Diabetes: Diabetes, Causes, Symptoms & Effects and How To Manage It For A Healthy, Successful Life

Table of Contents

Introduction

Chapter 1 Diabetes Causes and Symptoms

Chapter 2 Better Food Management to Reverse Your Diabetes

Chapter 3 Grains and Starchy Vegetables

Chapter 4 Healthy Fats

Chapter 5 Proteins

Chapter 6 Sugar and Desserts

Chapter 7 Exercise and Diabetic Management

Chapter 8 Supplementation and Medical Checkups

Chapter 9 Developing Habits to Manage Your Diabetes

Conclusion

Introduction

This book contains proven steps and strategies on how to manage or reverse your diabetes. Any person diagnosed with diabetes has a lot of questions on his or her mind: what diet should I follow? What lifestyle changes are needed? And various other questions.

Usually, doctors tell their patients to start to live a healthy lifestyle, which includes diet changes and physical activities. Until recently, doctors believed that once a patient has developed diabetes, he or she have to live with it for life and could anticipate one health condition after another, from kidney problems to worsening eyesight, high blood pressure, and heart problem.

This compassionate book based on the latest research demonstrates that managing or even reversing diabetes is possible with a healthy diet plan, regular exercise, additional supplements and positive mindset. This all-inclusive guide on diabetes is written in a clear, concise and down-to-earth language and include the causes, symptoms, and everything you have to do to reverse your diabetes.

Copyright 2016 by Lifestyledawn - All rights reserved.

Chapter 1 Diabetes Causes and Symptoms

What is Diabetes?

Diabetes is a serious health condition in which your body has a reduced ability to remove glucose from your blood and into its cells after consuming anything that contains carbohydrates. Your body uses various enzymes to transform the food that you eat. Food is broken down into macro and micro nutrients and used for different part of the body. For example, fat is needed for brain function and carbohydrates provide energy for your body.

Your body transforms carbohydrates into simpler forms knows as glucose or blood sugar. Glucose is released into the bloodstream to cope with immediate energy need or stored as fat for later use. Your body produces a hormone known as insulin to store and use glucose; insulin is produced in your pancreas. Your body needs insulin to get glucose from the bloodstream into the cells of the body. Insulin is released depending on the glucose presence in the blood. The insulin production tells your body cells to accept glucose as energy. This slowly diminishes glucose presence in the bloodstream and lead to decreased production of insulin.

Insulin resistance

Insulin resistance is a condition in which your body produces insulin but your body doesn't use it effectively. When your body develops insulin resistance, glucose accumulates in the bloodstream instead of being absorbed by the body cells. Leading to prediabetes or type 2 diabetes.

There are three different types of diabetes

- Type 1
- Type 2
- Gestational diabetes

Type 1 diabetes

Type 1 diabetes is mainly diagnosed in children and young adults. It is also known as juvenile diabetes. In type 1 diabetes, the body is unable to produce insulin. Young children can manage their condition with insulin therapy and other treatments. Only about 5% of diabetic patients have this form of diabetes. The exact cause of type 1 diabetes is still unknown, but scientists think that a **combination** of environmental and genetic susceptibility factors cause type 1 diabetes.

Type 2 diabetes

Type 2 diabetes is a condition where the body doesn't produce enough insulin or the body's cells don't react to insulin. This condition is called insulin resistance. Type 2 diabetic patients can control their illness by following a healthy diet, exercising regularly and regularly monitoring their blood glucose levels.

Gestational diabetes

Some women develop diabetes during pregnancy because they have high levels of glucose and their body is unable to produce enough insulin to absorb it. This is called gestational diabetes and affects nearly 18% women during pregnancy.

Shocking Statistics in the U.S.

- Data provided by the National Diabetes Report 2014, demonstrates that 29.1 million Americans or about 9.3% of the US population has diabetes and 86 million have developed pre-diabetes symptoms.
- The ratio children and adolescents with diabetes are alarming: 1 in 400.
- 11 million people who are 65 and older have diabetes
- Diabetes affects both men and women. 15.5 million men and 13.4 million women who are between 20 -50 have diabetes.
- Diabetes is one of the major causes of death and illness in the U.S. Diabetes close association with other major health problems such as heart disease, high blood pressure, stroke and cancer makes it deadly.

Factors that increase your type 2 diabetes risk:

Understanding why diabetes happens can help you to prevent diabetes:

- Obesity: If you are overweight or obese, your risk of developing type 2 diabetes is high. A body mass index (BMI) 30 or above is categorized as overweight or obese. Data provided by the National Institute of Diabetes and Digestive and Kidney Diseases shows that nearly 80% diabetic patients are obese or overweight. Fat accumulation around your abdomen area is especially dangerous because it releases chemicals that imbalance the body's metabolic and cardiovascular system. The fat around your belly also increases your risk of developing a variety of serious health conditions. Calculate your BMI if you are overweight or not.

- Physical Inactivity: According to the Archives of Internal Medicine, living a sedentary lifestyle can lead to diabetes, even if you are not overweight or obese. Alternatively, if you are obese or overweight, exercising and physical activity can lower your diabetes risk.

- Age: With age your risk of developing type 2 diabetes gets higher. This is because people tend to gain weight and avoid exercise when they get older.

- Genetics: If you have a close relative such as a parent, brother or sister with diabetes, your risk of diabetes is higher. Studies show that a child who has a parent with type 2 diabetes has a 30% chance of developing diabetes.

- Ethnicity: Studies show that African-Caribbean, black African, south Asian, and Chinese people are more likely to develop type 2 diabetes.

- Smoking: The smoke of the cigarettes increase inflammation in the body. So cigarette smokers are at greater risk of diabetes than nonsmokers. Researchers have shown that smoking raises blood glucose levels and deteriorate insulin resistance.

Low fiber diet: Your body can't break down fiber into glucose so fiber doesn't cause unstable blood sugar. Fiber rich food benefits the body a number of ways. Eating fiber rich foods lower the amount of insulin needed after you have eaten a meal or snack.

- Sugar rich beverages: Studies show that people who drink one or two sugar-rich beverages daily had a 26% higher risk of developing type 2 diabetes than people who drink them once monthly.

Diabetes Symptoms

Following are some usual symptoms of diabetes. But remember, some people have type 2 diabetes, but the symptoms are so mild that they are unnoticed.

- Blurry vision
- Urinating often
- Extreme fatigue

- Numbness, tingling or pain in the hands or feet
- Feeling very thirsty
- Cuts or bruises that are slow to heal
- Feeling very hungry
- Feeling sick
- Abdominal pain

Effects of diabetes on your body

- Dry and cracked skin
- Damaged blood vessels
- Lose of consciousness
- Stomach problems
- Foot problems
- Cataracts and Glaucoma
- Bacterial, Fungal and yeast infections
- Peripheral Neuropathy
- High blood pressure
- Heart disease
- Stroke

Chapter 2 Better Food Management to Reverse Your Diabetes

Follow a healthy eating plan if you have diabetes. A balanced and healthy eating plan can help you:

- Maintain a healthy body weight
- Maintain a healthy blood pressure
- Better manage your blood glucose levels
- Achieve target blood lipid or fat levels
- Slow down or even prevent the development of diabetes complications

If you have developed diabetes, then you should follow a guideline for consuming foods. Include food from the five food groups. This approach of eating will provide much-needed vitamins and nutrient you need to remain healthy and prevent other diseases such as heart disease and stroke.

To manage your diabetes

- Eat smaller but frequent meals throughout your day
- Follow a diet that is low in fat, especially saturated fat
- Eat snacks between your meals if you take diabetes tablets or insulin
- Remember, "one diet does not fit all". Everyone's needs are different.

Energy balance

Balancing the amount of food you eat with the amount of energy you burn through exercise and physical activity is important. Living an inactive life and eating too much can lead to weight gain. If you already have diabetes, then overweight or obesity can make it even more difficult to manage your diabetes. Furthermore, weight gain increases your risk of heart disease, stroke, and cancer.

As a diabetic patient, you can try a few different approaches to create a diabetes diet that keeps your blood glucose levels stable. There are mainly three different approaches for you to follow:

1. Carbohydrate Counting
2. The Plate Method
3. The Glycemic Index

Carbohydrate Counting

Carb counting or carbohydrate counting is an effective method to keep your blood glucose levels at a normal level. As the name suggests, carb counting helps you keep track of how many carbohydrates you eat daily.

How many carbohydrates?

Carbohydrate requirement varies from person to person. The right amount of carbohydrate depends on your activity/exercise levels and if you are taking any medications or not. Physically active people can eat more carb; however, inactive people have to eat less carbohydrate to keep their blood glucose stable. Taking 45 to 60 grams of carbohydrate per meal is a starting point for people who live a moderately active lifestyle. Lower or increase your carb intake depending on your activity level.

Foods that have Carbohydrate

- Starchy vegetables like potatoes, and peas
- Grains like barley, corn, rice and oatmeal
- Grain-based foods like cereal, bread, crackers, and pasta
- Milk and yogurt
- Fruit and fruit juice
- Soy products like veggie burgers, and dried beans like pinto beans
- Sweets and snack foods such as cake, candy, chips, sodas, juice drinks

Food labels will give you a good idea how much carbohydrate is in a food.

Each of the following foods contains 15 grams of carbohydrate:

- 1 small piece of fresh fruit (4 oz)
- 1/2 cup of canned or frozen fruit
- 1 slice of bread (1 oz) or 1 (6 inch) tortilla
- 1/2 cup of oatmeal
- 1/3 cup of pasta or rice
- 4-6 crackers
- 1/2 English muffin or hamburger bun
- 1/2 cup of black beans or starchy vegetable
- 1/4 of a large baked potato (3 oz)
- 2/3 cup of plain fat-free yogurt or sweetened with sugar substitutes
- 2 small cookies
- 2 inch square brownie or cake without frosting
- 1/2 cup ice cream or sherbet
- 1 Tbsp syrup, jam, jelly, sugar or honey
- 2 Tbsp light syrup
- 6 chicken nuggets
- 1/2 cup of casserole
- 1 cup of soup
- 1/4 serving of a medium french fry

The Plate Method

Create your plate method is an effective way to control your blood glucose levels, lose weight and prevent or even reverse diabetes. With this method, you fill your plate with grains, starchy foods, protein and non-starchy vegetables.

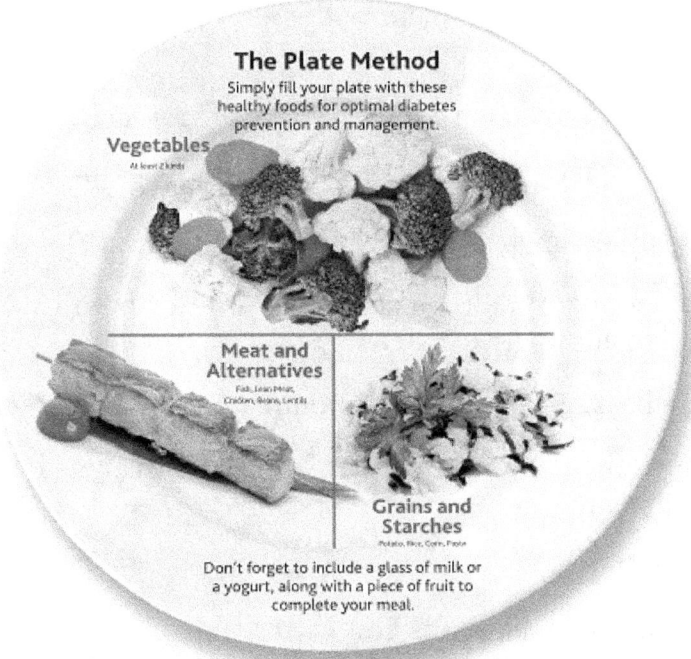

Simple rules to create your plate

- Just like the above picture divide your dinner plate according to food groups.
- Fill the biggest section with non-starchy vegetables.
- Fill one small section with starchy foods and grains.
- Fill the other small section with protein.
- Add a serving of dairy, a serving of fruit or both if your meal plan allows it.
- Choose healthy fats in small amounts
- Finish with a low-calorie drink like unsweetened tea, coffee or water.

The Glycemic Index

GI or glycemic index measures how carb rich foods raise blood glucose. Foods are judged based on how they match with a referee food. A high GI food raises blood glucose more than food that has a low GI. The glycemic index meal planning involves choosing foods that have a low or medium GI. You can eat mostly low and medium GI foods with a few high GI foods to help balance your meal. Fats and meats don't have GI because they don't contain carbohydrate.

Things that affect the GI of a food

Fiber and fats tend to lower the GI of a high GI food. Usually processed and cooked foods have a higher GI. Other factors that affect the GI of a food:

- Ripeness: Ripe fruit and vegetables have a higher GI
- Processed: Such as mashed potato has a higher GI than a whole baked potato, fruit juices have a higher GI than whole fruit and processed white bread have a higher GI than stone ground whole wheat bread.

- Cooking method: Longer cooking time raises GI in foods
- Variety: Longer variety tends to have lower GI, such as long-grain white rice has a lower GI than brown rice and short-grain white rice is higher GI than brown rice.

Examples of foods based on GI

Low GI Foods (55 or less)
- 100% stone-ground whole wheat or pumpernickel bread
- Oatmeal (rolled or steel-cut), oat bran, muesli
- Pasta, converted rice, barley, bulgar
- Sweet potato, corn, yam, lima/butter beans, peas, legumes and lentils
- Most fruits, non-starchy vegetables and carrots

Medium GI (56-69)
- Whole wheat, rye and pita bread
- Quick oats
- Brown, wild or basmati rice, couscous

High GI (70 or more)
- White bread or bagel
- Corn flakes, puffed rice, bran flakes, instant oatmeal
- Shortgrain white rice, rice pasta, macaroni and cheese from mix
- Russet potato, pumpkin
- Pretzels, rice cakes, popcorn, saltine crackers
- melons and pineapple

Choosing the best method

Every person is different and there is no universal diet plan for every diabetic patient. The important thing for you to follow a meal plan that goes with your lifestyle, personal preferences and helps accomplish goals for blood pressure, cholesterol, blood glucose, triglycerides levels and weight management. Studies show that both the type and the amount of carbohydrate in food affect blood glucose levels. Studies also show that total carbohydrate in food is a better predictor of blood glucose response than the glycemic index of food.

Most diabetic patients find some type of carbohydrate counting very useful. The type of carbohydrate affects blood glucose, so use the glycemic index to "fine-tune" your blood glucose management. Meaning combining carbohydrate counting with GI to get added benefit.

Chapter 3 Grains and Starchy Vegetables

As a diabetic patient, whole grains are your best choice. Whole grains are rich in fiber, vitamins, minerals and phytochemicals. When buying foods, reading labels is important. It will help you understand if you are making the right choices or not.

Nutrition facts label

When buying packaged foods, you can use the nutrition facts label to guide you. Check the serving size first, then the total carbohydrate. Even if food is labeled as no sugar added, sugar-free, or reduced sugar, it can still contain carbohydrate because sugar is only one form of carbohydrate that affects your blood glucose levels. Read the Nutrition Facts Panel to know the complete amount of carbohydrate.

① **Start Here** →

Nutrition Facts
Serving Size 1 cup (228g)
Servings Per Container 2

② **Check Calories**

Amount Per Serving
Calories 250   Calories from Fat 110

	% Daily Value*
Total Fat 12g	18%
Saturated Fat 3g	15%
Trans Fat 3g	
Cholesterol 30mg	10%
Sodium 470mg	20%
Total Carbohydrate 31g	10%

③ **Limit these Nutrients**

⑥ **Quick Guide to % DV**

Dietary Fiber 0g	0%
Sugars 5g	
Protein 5g	
Vitamin A	4%
Vitamin C	2%
Calcium	20%
Iron	4%

• **5% or less is Low**

• **20% or more is High**

④ **Get Enough of these Nutrients**

⑤ **Footnote**

* Percent Daily Values are based on a 2,000 calorie diet. Your Daily Values may be higher or lower depending on your calorie needs.

	Calories:	2,000	2,500
Total Fat	Less than	65g	80g
Sat Fat	Less than	20g	25g
Cholesterol	Less than	300mg	300mg
Sodium	Less than	2,400mg	2,400mg
Total Carbohydrate		300g	375g
Dietary Fiber		25g	30g

Food Labels reading guideline

- Read the serving size. All the information on the label is related to the serving of the food.
- Read the grams of total carbohydrate. Total carbohydrate on the label includes starch, fiber, and sugar.
- If you want to lose weight, then look at the calories.
- To lower your risk of heart disease and stroke, the saturated and trans fat content is important. Choose products with a lower amount of saturated and trans fats per serving.
- If you have a high blood pressure problem, then look at the sodium content. Choose foods with less sodium.

If you don't have time and patience reading the entire label, then just look at the total carbohydrate in a specific food. The total carbohydrate includes sugar, sugar alcohols, starch, and fiber. Reading total carbohydrate is extremely helpful because it includes both starch and sugar.

What is whole grain

A whole grain is an entire grain, including the endosperm (starchy part), bran and germ. Wheat is the most popular grain in the US. Examples of whole grain wheat products include 100% whole wheat bread, crackers, tortillas, and pasta. Finding whole grain food can be difficult because often foods contain a small amount of whole grain, but vaguely says it contains whole grains on the front of the package. When buying grains and cereals, read the ingredient list carefully. Try to find the following sources of whole grains on top of the ingredient list, when buying:

- Wild rice
- Brown rice
- Whole rye

- Bulgur
- Whole grain corn/corn meal
- Popcorn
- Whole grain barley
- Whole wheat flour
- Sorghum
- Millet

- Triticale
- Buckwheat
- Buckwheat flour
- Quinoa
- Wild farro

Most bread, cereals, rolls, and crackers labeled as "containing" or "made with" whole grain don't show whole grain as the first ingredient. Reading labels is extremely important to find the perfect food and food product for you.

Starchy Vegetables

Starchy vegetables offer you fiber, vitamins and minerals and don't have added sugar, fat or sodium.

Try a variety such as:

- Green peas
- Potato
- Parsnip
- Pumpkin
- Butternut squash
- Acorn squash

Often people think corn as a vegetable, but it is actually a grain.

Dried beans, legumes, peas, and lentils

Eat dried beans several times a week. They offer you fiber, protein, vitamins and minerals.

- Dried peas, such as split and black-eyed

- Fat-free refried beans
- Dried beans such as lima, black, and pinto
- Lentils
- Vegetarian baked beans

Chapter 4 Healthy Fats

Fats are full with energy. Eating excessive fat can lead to quick weight gain and make it difficult to manage blood glucose levels. Your body needs a small amount of healthy fat for proper functioning, so choose your fats wisely.

Saturated Fat

Saturated fats tend to raise your LDL or bad cholesterol levels so limit your saturated fat intake. Animal foods like full-fat milk, butter, cheese and fatty meats are high in saturated fat. Vegetable fats that are saturated include coconut products (such as coconut milk, cream, and copha) and palm oil (found in snack foods, convenience foods and as solid cooking fats).

Follow these rules to lower your saturated fat consumption:

- Eat low-fat or non-fat milk, yogurt, custard, ice-cream and cheese
- Eat lean meats and trim any fat off before cooking
- Remove the skin from poultry such as duck, chicken before cooking
- Avoid using coconut milk, coconut cream, copra, butter, lard, cream, sour cream, dripping and hard cooking margarine
- Limit puddings, cakes, pastries, cream biscuits and chocolate
- Limit prepackaged cakes, biscuits, savory packet snacks, frozen and convenience meals
- Limit the use of processed deli meats (such as chicken loaf, salami, sausages, lunch meat, etc.)
- Avoid fried takeaway foods such as battered fish, fried chicken, chips and choose grilled fish and BBQ chicken (without the skin) instead.

- Avoid pastries, pies and sausage rolls
- Avoid dressings and creamy sauces and use soy, tomato or other low-fat ingredients.
- Limit creamy style soups.

Trans fats

- Baked goods, processed snacks, stick margarine and shortening all contain trans fats. Completely avoid all of them.
- Cholesterol: High-fat animal proteins and high-fat dairy products contain cholesterol. Food items such as shellfish, egg yolks, liver and other organ meats all contain cholesterol. Ideally, you should eat maximum 300 mg of cholesterol daily.

Sodium

For healthy people, less than 2,300 mg of sodium daily is recommended. But for high blood pressure patients, around 1300 to 1500 mg is recommended.

Polyunsaturated and monounsaturated fats

Eating small amounts of monounsaturated and polyunsaturated fats can help ensure that your body get much-needed essential fatty acids and vitamins.

Polyunsaturated fats include:

- Oily fishes such as mackerel, herring, salmon, tuna, and sardine
- Safflower, soybean, sunflower, corn, grapeseed, cottonseed, and sesame oils
- Polyunsaturated margarines

Monounsaturated fats include:

- Avocado, Canola and olive oils
- Some margarines

Nuts, nut butter, and seeds contain a combination of monounsaturated and polyunsaturated fat.

Few simple ideas for enjoying healthy fats

- Eat linseed bread with a little canola margarine
- Eat a handful of unsalted nuts as a snack or add them to your salad or stir-fry
- Eat avocados with salad or use avocado spread on sandwiches
- Stir-fry vegetables and meats in a small amount of canola oil or use cooking spray
- Use olive oil, lemon juice or vinegar as a salad dressing
- Sprinkle sesame seeds on your steamed vegetables
- Eat fish, at least three times weekly because they contain healthy oil omega-3.
- Avoid battered, deep-fried and crumbed foods
- Use non-stick pan for roasting, grilling and microwaving

Chapter 5 Proteins

Your body needs protein for growth and repair. A moderate amount of protein does not raise blood glucose levels. But avoid eating too much protein rich food because your body converts excess protein to glucose.

Best choices of protein for you:

- Chicken and other poultry
- Fish and seafood
- Cheese and eggs
- Plant-based proteins

1. Poultry: Choose poultry such as chicken, turkey and Cornish hen without skin for less saturated fat and cholesterol. Game birds such as goose, dove, duck, pheasant.

2. Fish and seafood: Eat fish twice weekly. Eat fishes that are high in omega-3 fatty acids like mackerel, tuna, salmon, trout, herring, sardines. Other beneficial fish and seafood include haddock, halibut, tilapia, crab, scallops, oysters, shrimp, etc.

3. Cheese and Eggs: This section includes egg whites and egg substitutes, cottage cheese, reduced-fat cheese.

4. Plant-based proteins provide fiber, quality protein, and healthy fat. Eat:

- Soy nuts
- Edamame
- Beans such as kidney, black and pinto
- Hummus and falafel
- Bean products like refined beans and baked beans

- Meatless beef crumble, chicken nuggets, bacon, burgers, hot dogs and sausage
- Tempeh, tofu
- Lentils such as green, yellow or brown
- Peas such as split or black-eyed peas
- Nuts and spreads like cashew butter, almond butter or peanut butter

- Beef, lamb, pork, and veal

If you decide to eat them, choose the leanest options, which are:

- Beef jerky
- Beef parts trimmed of fat, including rib, rump roast, chuck, cubed, sirloin, round, porterhouse, tenderloin, T-bone steak
- Lamb: leg, chop or roast
- Pork: ham, tenderloin, Canadian bacon, center loin chops
- Organ meats: kidney, heart, liver

Game meat includes: buffalo, ostrich, venison, rabbit

Chapter 6 Sugar and Desserts

As a diabetic patient if is best if you try a piece of fresh fruit or fruit salad. Whenever you decide it's treat time, keep your portions small. However, don't get discouraged because having diabetes doesn't mean you have to avoid everything sweet. With a little planning, you can enjoy sweet treats now and then.

Thoughts on sugar

Sugar rich drinks contribute to weight gain and accelerates your risk of developing type 2 diabetes. This is why the American Diabetes Association and other health organizations recommend that people limit or avoid sugar-sweetened beverages to prevent diabetes. Build your diet plan based on vegetables, whole grains, fruit, beans, fish, lean meats, non-fat dairy and eat a small serving of sweets occasionally.

Introducing sweets in your meal plan

Following sweeteners have a high amount of calories and carbohydrates:

o Table sugar also is known as sucrose or white sugar
o Beet sugar
o Agave nectar
o Turbinado
o Rice syrup or brown rice syrup
o Raw sugar
o Sugar cane syrup
o Maple syrup
o Cane sugar
o Molasses

- Fructose
- Honey
- Powdered sugar
- Confectioners sugar
- Coconut palm sugar

Occasionally, when you decide to eat a sweet treat, substitute it with other carb-containing foods in your meals and snacks. Following are some carb containing foods:

- Corn
- Bread
- Peas
- Rice
- Tortillas
- Yogurt
- Potatoes
- Crackers
- Milk
- Fruit
- Juice

When eating sweets, cut back on other carb-containing foods. For example, you want to eat cupcakes after lunch and your lunch is a double bread turkey sandwich. Take following steps to make the substitution:

- Identify carb in your meal, and bread is the obvious one.
- Change the regular bread with two slices of low-carb bread, (1/2 carb) and have the cupcake.
- This way, your total calorie consumption remains the same.

Chapter 7 Exercise and Diabetic Management

Regular physical exercise helps you to lower blood glucose, including:

- Exercise improves insulin sensitivity. With improved insulin sensitivity, your body cells are able to better utilize any available insulin during and after activity.

- Your muscles contract during exercise and it stimulates another mechanism, which is unrelated to insulin. This separate mechanism allows your cells to collect glucose from the bloodstream and use it for energy even if insulin is not available.

The above are short-term benefits of exercise. Exercise also offers you other long-term benefits.

Mainly two types of physical activity/ exercises are important for diabetic patients:

- Aerobic exercise
- Strength training

Aerobic Exercise

Aerobic exercise relieves stress, makes your heart and bones strong, improves blood circulation, helps your body use insulin better and lower your risk for heart disease by reducing blood glucose levels and blood pressure and improving good cholesterol levels. Experts recommend 30 minutes of moderate or vigorous intensity aerobic exercise 5 days weekly or 150 minutes of exercise per week. Try not to spend two days without exercising.

Start with 10 or even 5 minutes daily and increase your activity as you get used to exercising. If you are busy and can't find 30 minutes for exercise, then divide your exercise time 10-minute sessions and make things easy for you. If you want to lose weight, then 60 minutes of aerobic exercise daily is recommended.

Here are a few examples of aerobic activities:

- Low-impact aerobics
- Brisk walking
- Jogging/running
- Dancing
- Bicycling
- Moderate-to-heavy gardening

- Hiking
- Ice-skating or roller-skating
- Stair climbing
- Rowing
- Swimming or water aerobics
- Cross-country skiing
- Playing tennis

Strength Training

Resistance training or strength training makes your body more sensitive to insulin and helps lower blood glucose. Also, strength training helps to build and maintain strong muscles and bones and lower your risk of osteoporosis when you age. With more muscle tissue, you burn more calories, even when you are resting. In addition to aerobic exercise, experts recommend some type of strength training at least twice weekly. Following are some examples of strength training:

- Using resistance bands
- Lifting weights
- Weight machines or free weights at the gym
- Classes that involve strength training
- Pushups, squats, lunges, sit-ups, and planks
- Heavy gardening

Examples of weekly 150 minutes of moderate activity

- 35 minutes of jogging, 3 times weekly. Weight lifting twice a week.
- 30 minutes of brisk walking, 5 times weekly. Resistance bands 2 times weekly.

- 30 minutes of brisk walk, twice weekly. 45 minutes of tennis doubles, twice weekly. Weight machines twice weekly.

- 30 minutes of the stationary bike twice weekly. 30 minutes of lawn mowing one afternoon, heavy gardening twice weekly. 60 minutes of dancing one evening, weekly.

Chapter 8 Supplementation and Medical Checkups

Studies have shown that dietary supplements can help you to manage your diabetes.

Multivitamin

The main argument in favor of taking a multivitamin daily is that often people don't follow a balanced diet. So if you are following a balanced diet, then you don't need any multivitamin.

Magnesium

Magnesium plays an important role in your blood sugar regulation. Several studies have shown that adequate amount of dietary magnesium consumption is associated with a reduced risk of diabetes. Preferably you should get your magnesium from natural sources, such as spinach, artichokes, whole grain bread, brown rice, avocados, and nuts.

Vitamin D

Vitamin D deficiency is associated with higher rates of autoimmune diseases, bone disease, mood disorders, cardiovascular disease and some types of cancer. Vitamin D deficiency has been identified as one of the root causes of insulin resistance and diabetes because vitamin D effect pancreatic cell function. Mid-day sun exposure is one of the easiest ways to get your vitamin D. Food sources of vitamin D include: Salmon, tuna, sardines, trout, halibut, swordfish, rockfish, oysters, egg yolks, shiitake mushrooms, Swiss cheese and fortified foods such as milk, and yogurts.

Omega -3 Fats

Omega -3 lowers inflammation and improve insulin resistance. Take omega-3 fats from wild-caught fish, grass-fed meat, dark green leafy vegetables, walnuts, hemp seeds, chia seeds, and flaxseeds.

You can eat healthy foods and exercise regularly to control your blood sugar levels. However, regular health checkups and tests are also important. These visits to your doctor will give you a chance to:

- Ask question about your blood sugar levels
- An opportunity to learn more about diabetes and additional steps you should take to control your blood sugar
- Making sure that you are taking your diabetic medications correctly

Do medical exams every 3 to 6 months. During your exam, your doctor should check your blood pressure, feet, and weight.

Hemoglobin A1c tests

Do hemoglobin A1c tests after every three months. A1c tests show how you are managing your blood sugar levels. The normal level is less than 6%, so your aim should be keeping it under 7%.

Chapter 9 Developing Habits to Manage Your Diabetes

Following habits will help you lose weight, improve insulin sensitivity and reverse diabetes.

- Learn how your body works: Losing weight is not an easy task. The human body doesn't like sudden reduction in calorie intake because it indicates the body an impending food shortage. So cut calories in small portions, such as start to drink calorie-free beverages, limit eating out, etc.

- Change your attitude: Just remember, even though you have diabetes, you are not a failure. Following these strategies will help you lose weight and reverse diabetes. Successful people see lapses as an opportunity to learn, not a sign of weakness.

- Keep a food journal: Various studies have shown that keeping a food journal is extremely helpful. It keeps people accountable for what they are eating. Use a notebook and keep a detailed record of your food and beverage consumption, the time and the amount of food you eat throughout the day. A food journal will provide you revealing information about your food habit and it will keep your diet goals in front of you. Every time you write in your notebook, it will act as a reminder of what you are trying to achieve.

- Avoid overeating at night: Timing and the amount of food you eat during each meal is also important. For people who are obese and developed diabetes, a familiar pattern often appears where food consumption accelerates as the day goes on. Avoid overeating at night and balance your meals throughout the day. Eat three main meals: breakfast, lunch and dinner and two snacks in between meals.

- Budget time for self-care: Humans are designed to be opportunistic eaters. This approach worked well for our hunter-gatherer ancestors, but today we are overexposed to carb rich unhealthy foods. We are living an extremely busy life and making time for healthy eating and exercise seems impossible. However, to manage or even reverse your diabetic, you have to resist the temptation of eating easily available calorie rich foods and make time for physical activity. Create a pie chart of all the activities that demands your attention. The chart will include your family, work, pets, friends, hobbies and other things that are important to you. To live a healthy life, you need to allocate time for self-care, such as: buying healthy foods, preparing, and cooking, physical activity, 6-8 hours of sleep, and managing stress.

- Manage your hunger: Remaining long period without eating any food is one of the main reasons we overeat. Use an imaginary scale (0-10) to calculate your hunger, where 0 is no hunger and 10 is starving. Eat when your hunger is 5 or 6 and avoid overeating.
- Manage your expectations: Making constructive changes to your lifestyle and diet is difficult. So manage your expectations to make things easier for you:
    - Pay attention to what is your body is trying to tell you
    - Set a temporary goal and focus on getting through a single day
    - Change is hard, so go easy on yourself
    - You can't change the past, but you can learn from it
    - Appreciate the positive feedback you get from eating healthier and exercising regularly.
    - Plan your meals in advance. This approach will help you make better choices. Focus on the foods that you can eat. Don't bring high-risk foods in your house.
    - Eat enough good foods so that there is no room for bad foods.

Don't try to do it alone: Ask for support. Your partner, spouse, other family members, friend or exercise buddy can be an invaluable asset. If you are a group person, then join a group that is trying to manage diabetic together. Many find guidance from a registered dietitian useful. Go to the Academy of Nutrition and Dietetics official website **www.eatright.org** to find a dietitian near you. The website will also give you valuable information on how you can manage your diet.

Conclusion

As a diabetic patient, patience is perhaps the most important skill for long-term success. Remember, time is needed for your body to get used to eating less carb-rich foods and for you to feel the positive effects of exercise. With practice and patience, you can manage or even reverse your diabetes.

www.ingramcontent.com/pod-product-compliance
Lightning Source LLC
Chambersburg PA
CBHW071830200526
45169CB00018B/1302